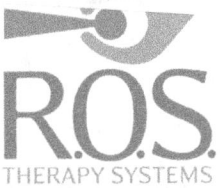

R.O.S. THERAPY SYSTEMS

R.O.S. Therapy Systems Presents:

Caregiver Activity Lesson Plans
Beer and Wine Activities

Word Scramble

Code Breakers

Word Search

Crossword

Trivia

How Much Do You Know About?

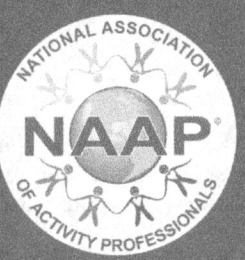

NATIONAL ASSOCIATION OF ACTIVITY PROFESSIONALS

NAAP

Scott Silknitter

VOLUME 1

Caregiver Activity Lesson Plans

How Much Do You Know About Wine and Beer

This edition of the *Caregiver Activity Lesson Plans* features some of the favorite activities of leading Activity Professionals from around the United States. Activity Professionals are the quality of life experts that focus on the social side of long-term care and design individual programs for every resident, client or participant they work with. We have adapted those activities to make a booklet of one-to-one activities that can be used by any caregiver in any setting.

About NAAP

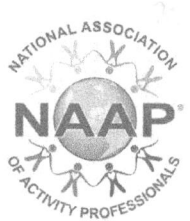

Since 1981, the National Association of Activity Professionals (NAAP) has led the way for activities for residents in long-term care settings. Whether it is lobbying for and setting standards, educating members and the general public or promoting quality of life initiatives for those in any institutional setting, NAAP has been the driving force behind person-centered and person-appropriate social care.

About R.O.S. Therapy Systems

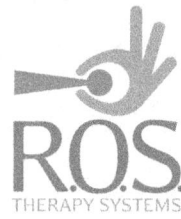

R.O.S. Therapy Systems began as a backyard project to help one family with their quality of life during a 25-year fight with Parkinson's and dementia. The company has grown into a trusted partner for Family Caregivers, Home Care Agencies, Adult Day Centers, Assisted Living Facilities and Skilled Nursing Facilities.

ISBN   978-1518603778

Published by
R.O.S. Therapy Systems, L.L.C.
Greensboro, NC
888-352-9788
www.ROSTherapySystems.com

How to use an Activity Lesson Plan:

An Activity Lesson Plan should be ever-changing. It is meant to be written on and to note the changes you may have made from the original plan so that the next person working with the participant can follow your modifications with the goal of recreating positive experiences.

Date: Document the date the activity is used with the participant

Activity Name: Name of the activity being performed

Objective: To provide meaningful, purposeful activities that will engage

Materials: Suggested materials and resources to use with this activity

Prerequisite Skills: Skills and abilities a person should possess for this activity

Activity Outline: Step-by-step instructions to complete the activity

Evaluation: A thorough evaluation is the most important part of the Lesson Plan. When conducting an activity with the participant, record any verbal cues, assistance, or modifications to incorporate into the activity. It is also helpful to include the participants response to the program.

Note programs that are successful at distracting or eliminating a negative behavior (diversion activities). Encourage family members and caregivers to use the evaluation section and also leave tips. Don't waste time recreating the wheel of knowledge. Pass on the information so everyone presents the activity in the same way with the same modifications and cueing, in order to achieve the same positive outcomes.

** A leader must be present at all times when conducting the activities contained in this book.

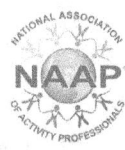

Adapting an Activity Lesson Plan

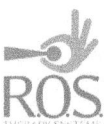

Every person has his or her own unique physical and cognitive abilities and needs. How that person responds to an activity will dictate how the leader will continue to modify or adapt an Activity Lesson Plan to meet an individual participants needs and abilities – now and in the future.

It is up to the leader to determine modifications to any Activity Lesson Plan so an activity is person-centered and person-appropriate. The following is an example of modifying an activity:

Butterfly Craft

You know that the participant loves butterflies. You decide to use an Activity Lesson Plan based on a butterfly craft. Depending on the participants physical and cognitive level, you will determine what adjustments have to be made. Here are examples of four functional levels and how your butterfly activity may be modified:

- Level 1: Coffee Filter Butterfly Craft: Take a coffee filter and paint it with watercolor paint. When it dries, pinch the center together and tie a pipe cleaner around the center in the shape of a butterfly body. Make two antennas out of the pipe cleaners.

- Level 2: Color pictures of butterflies

- Level 3: Look at the pictures and discuss butterflies together

- Level 4: The leader shows pictures of butterflies to the participant

To ensure the participant reaps the benefits of being engaged, please adapt any and all activities to the participants functional level.

The leader should read all step-by-step directions of an Activity Outline before beginning an activity with a participant. The step-by-step directions are general guidelines for the leader to use, and potentially modify, in order to help the participant successfully engage in the chosen activity.

Thank you for using this edition of Caregiver Activity Lesson Plans

R.O.S. Therapy Systems offers several *Caregiver Activity Lesson Plan* books. We have amassed hundreds of Activity Lesson Plans so there is something for everyone:

- Craft Activities
- Gardening Activities
- Outdoor Activities

- Holiday Activities
- Games
- Science Activities

- Activities for Men
- Baking Activities
- Art Activities

- Music Activities
- Verbal Communication Skills Activities
- Computer Activities

Please check www.ROSTherapySystems.com or www.therosstore.com to see a complete list of available *Caregiver Activity Lesson Plans* books. With new books being published regularly, please check back often.

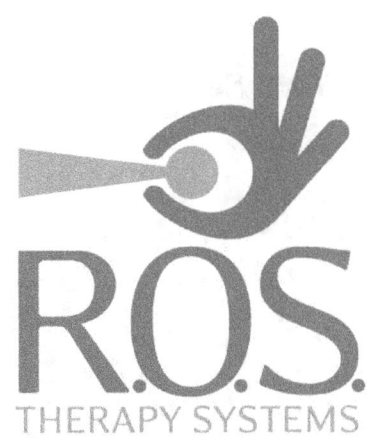

If we can help in any other way, please contact us directly at 888-352-9788

Caregiver Activity Lesson Plans
How Much Do You Know About:
Beer and Wine

Table of Contents

Caregiver Activity Lesson Plans
How Much Do You Know About:
Beer and Wine

Table of Contents

Activity Lesson Plans

Wine, Beer and Bartending Trivia

.

Wine, Beer and Bartending Trivia

- The following pages contain basic templates that can be used by anyone. The leader must allow for the participant to be successful.

- The leader should read all step-by-step directions of an Activity Outline before beginning an activity with a participant. The step-by-step directions are general guidelines for the leader/caregiver to use and potentially modify in order to help the participant successfully engage in the chosen activity.

- The leader must always be present when engaging the participant in an activity.

- The leader must take all necessary and reasonable precautions to ensure the safety of the participant.

- The leader should have necessary materials ready and prepared prior to the beginning of the activity.

- To ensure that the participant reaps the benefits of being engaged, please adapt any and all activities to the participants functional level.

Program Name: Wine and Beer Trivia   **Date:** _____

Leader: _____   **Time:** _____

Objective:

- Stimulate cognitive functioning
- Increase self-worth and improve self-esteem
- Increase socialization
- Foster friendship, laughter and closeness
- Provide a sense of accomplishment
- Stimulate memory
- Have some fun!

Materials:

- Flat surface for participant to write on
- Templates on the following pages provided
- Pen, pencil or high lighter

Note: If a participant is in a bed, recliner or wheelchair, consider using the R.O.S. Multi-Purpose Board Insert and the R.O.S. Legacy™ System Console available at R.O.S. Therapy Systems (www.therosstore.com) as an option for a flat surface to allow the participant the opportunity to fully engage in this activity.

Prerequisite Skills:

Every person has his or her own unique physical/cognitive abilities and needs. How a participant responds to an activity will dictate how the caregiver will modify or adapt a Lesson Plan to meet individual client needs and abilities – now and in the future.

Program Name: Wine and Beer Trivia   **Date:** _____

Leader: _____   **Time:** _____

Activity Outline:

The leader explains to the participant that they will be playing a trivia game.

1. Use the following templates to enjoy trivia based on topics of interest.

Option 1: Based on the participants abilities, the participant completes the activity on their own.

Option 2: Based on the participants abilities, the leader assists with finding answers.

Option 3: Based on the participants abilities, the leader and the participant have a discussion based on words and topics included in this activity.

Evaluation:

Red Wine – Trivia

1. Which term refers to the geographic origin of the grapes used to make a particular wine?

   _____

2. Which term means "soil" in French and refers to the geographical and physical environment in which the grapes used to make a wine were grown?

   _____

3. Beaujolais, Bordeaux, and Burgundy are wine-growing regions in which country?

   _____

4. This medium to full-bodied red wine is high in tannins, and its flavor is often described as having hints of blackberry, plum, oak, and chocolate.

   _____

5. What is the optimal temperature for storing red wine?

   _____

6. At what temperature should red wine be served?

   _____

7. What are the four steps of tasting red wines?

   _____

Red Wine – Trivia

8. What three characteristics should you look for when tasting red wine?

   _____

9. What is the name for the wine drips on the side of your glass that you might see after swirling your wine?

   _____

10. Where do flavors in red wines such as vanilla, caramel, molasses, and toasted notes come from?

    _____

11. Terms like vegetal, earthy, and floral are used to describe which feature of red wine?

    _____

12. Why would a wine be called "flabby"?

    _____

13. Which country is associated with Chianti?

    _____

14. What is the term for the plastic or foil covering the cork and neck part of a wine bottle?

    _____

Red Wine – Trivia

15. Which versatile wine grape originally came from Croatia but is now grown almost exclusively in California?

_____

16. Which red wine grape requires nearly perfect growing conditions to produce a good quality wine?

_____

17. Which region of France is known for excellent Syrahs?

_____

18. Which country is best known for its Shiraz?

_____

19. What is special about Château de Goulaine, Barone Ricasoli, Schloss Johanisberg, and Schloss Vollrads?

_____

20. During which part of the winemaking process are the lees steeped to extract tannins, phenol compounds, and the fruit flavors that characterize a wine?

_____

Red Wine – Trivia

(answers)

1. Appellation
2. Terroir
3. France
4. Cabernet Sauvignon
5. Red wine should be stored at 55 degrees.
6. Red wine should be between 60 to 65 degrees to serve.
7. Eyeball, Swirl, Sniff, and Sip
8. Body, quality, and texture
9. Legs or tears
10. They come from the barrels in which the wines are fermented and aged.
11. Bouquet
12. Wines without enough acids are called flabby.
13. Italy
14. Capsule
15. Zinfandel
16. Pinot Noir
17. The Northern Rhone Valley
18. Australia
19. They are four of the oldest wineries in the world.
20. Maceration

White Wine – Trivia

1. What is considered the best temperature at which to serve white wine?

   _____

2. Do white wines become paler or darker in color as they age?

   _____

3. What are the world's three most planted white wine grapes?

   _____

4. How many white wine varieties can you name?

   _____

5. What region in Germany is known for its world-class Rieslings?

   _____

6. What are Asti, Cava, Champagne, and Prosecco?

   _____

7. Smoky, toasted bread, orange blossom, and rose are words used to describe what about a white wine?

   _____

White Wine – Trivia

8. Is white wine that has less than four grams of residual sugar per liter considered very dry, sour, or flabby?

   _____

9. This region in Italy produces Soave and Prosecco.

   _____

10. If you wanted a dry white wine with dinner, would you choose a Pinot grigio or a Prosecco?

    _____

11. What is added to white wine during a second fermentation to make champagne?

    _____

12. "Liebfraumilch," a semi-sweet white wine, translates to "beloved lady's milk" in which language?

    _____

13. The science, production, and study of grapes is____?

    _____

14. A glass for drinking white wine has more of a u-shaped bowl than a glass for red wine. True or False?

    _____

White Wine – Trivia

15. What is the name for the kind of glass that you would use when drinking sparkling wine or champagne?

   _____

16. White wine can be made from either red or white grapes. True or False?

   _____

17. Contrary to popular myth, Dom Pérignon did not discover the method for making champagne. Who was he?

   _____

18. Which two types of wine grapes go into making Dom Pérignon champagne?

   _____

19. If your white wine tastes a little grassy, what type of wine are you most likely drinking?

   _____

20. What is "Hárslevelű" in Hungarian, "Lipovina" in Slovak, "Feuille de Tilleul" in French, and "Lindenblättriger" in German?

   _____

White Wine – Trivia
(answers)

1. Between 50 and 55 degrees Farenheit
2. They become darker.
3. Airén, Chardonnay, and Ugni blanc
4. Chardonnay, Sauvignon blanc, Sémillon, Moscato, Pinot grigio or Pinot gris, Gewürztraminer, and Riesling are the main types of white wine.
5. Mosel
6. They are all sparkling white wines.
7. Its aroma
8. Very dry
9. Veneto
10. Pinot grigio
11. Yeast and rock sugar
12. German
13. Viticulture
14. True
15. Flute
16. True
17. He was a monk and cellar master at the Benedictine abbey in Hautvillers, France.
18. Pinot noir and Chardonnay
19. Sauvignon blanc
20. This is the name of a white wine grape used to make Tokaji and other dessert wines. The name refers to the "lime tree leaf."

Beer – Trivia

1. What are the key ingredients in making beer?

   _____

2. What is the first step in brewing beer?

   _____

3. Hard water is best for making what kind of beer?

   _____

4. Soft water is best for making what kind of beer?

   _____

5. The oldest working brewery is the Benedictine Weihenstephan Brewery. Where is it located?

   _____

6. A modern brewery that makes a limited amount of beer is called a …?

   _____

7. What type of beer is made from top-fermenting yeast?

   _____

Beer – Trivia

8. The sugars that result after the mashing process are known as ...?

   _____

9. This kind of beer from Germany is very dark and has a high alcohol content.

   _____

10. Beer that is dispensed from a keg is called ...?

    _____

11. In Germany, you'll likely drink your beer from a stein, and in Ireland your beer will probably come in a ...?

    _____

12. Steam beer was the first style of beer to come from which country?

    _____

13. Which was the first national beer brand in the U.S.?

    _____

14. What is zythology?

    _____

Beer – Trivia

15. Which is the oldest and largest American-owned brewery operating today? Where is it?

   _____

16. What is the most expensive beer in the world, and where would you have to go to get it?

   _____

17. Maine made an exception to its law prohibiting the sale of beer before 6 a.m. on Sundays when which holiday fell on a Sunday in 2013?

   _____

18. Which country has the most individual beer brands?

   _____

19. Which President signed a bill in 1978 that legalized home production of small amounts of beer?

   _____

20. Anchor Steam Beer is the oldest craft beer in America. In which California city is it made?

   _____

Beer – Trivia

(answers)

1. Water, barley, wheat, yeast, flavoring or hops
2. Mashing the barley
3. Stout
4. Pale lager or pilsner
5. Bavaria, Germany
6. Microbrewery or craft brewery
7. Pale ale
8. Wort
9. Dopplebock
10. Draught or draft
11. Tankard
12. United States
13. Budweiser
14. The study of beer and beer making
15. D.G. Yuengling & Son in Pottsville, PA
16. Vielle Bon Secours; Beirdrome in London
17. St. Patrick's Day
18. Belgium
19. Jimmy Carter
20. San Francisco

Bartender Trivia

1. Gin is made with berries from what plant?

    _____

2. This mixer is most often used with gin.

    _____

3. The name of this spirit is a Russian word meaning "little water."

    _____

4. Which spirit comes in both white and dark varieties?

    _____

5. Which spirit originated in the Scottish Highlands?

    _____

6. This is said to be the national spirit of Mexico.

    _____

7. If you mix gin, lemon juice, sugar and water, you are making which cocktail?

    _____

Bartender Trivia

8. How should a "neat" drink be served?

   _____

9. If someone orders a shot, they might also order what to drink right afterwards?

   _____

10. A daiquiri without alcohol is called a what?

    _____

11. After a day of skiing, someone who likes butter and cinnamon might order this to warm up with.

    _____

12. This kind of cherry is used as a drink garnish.

    _____

13. This Kentucky whiskey is at least 51% corn.

    _____

14. Which liqueur has a distinctive almond flavor?

    _____

Bartender Trivia

15. The theory and practice of bartending is known as?

   _____

16. This glass is designed to conserve the champagne bubbles inside.

   _____

17. What is a stick with a round end used to crush sugar?

   _____

18. A margarita might have this on its rim?

   _____

19. A martini made with a cocktail onion is called a what?

   _____

20. What is the name for a small cup used to measure out spirits for a cocktail?

   _____

Bartender Trivia

(answers)

1. Juniper
2. Tonic
3. Vodka
4. Rum
5. Whiskey
6. Tequila
7. Tom Collins
8. Without ice and a mixer
9. Chaser
10. Virgin
11. Hot Buttered Rum
12. Maraschino
13. Bourbon
14. Amaretto
15. Mixology
16. Flute
17. Muddler
18. Salt
19. Gibson
20. Jigger

Activity Lesson Plans

Wine, Beer and Bartending Word Scramble

Wine, Beer and Bartending Word Scramble

- The following pages contain basic templates that can be used with anyone. The leader must allow for the participant to be successful.

- The leader should read all step-by-step directions of an Activity Outline before beginning an activity with a participant. The step-by-step directions are general guidelines for the leader/ caregiver to use and potentially modify in order to help the participant successfully engage in the chosen activity.

- The leader must always be present when engaging the participant in an activity.

- The leader must take all necessary and reasonable precautions to ensure the safety of the participant.

- The leader should have necessary materials ready and prepared prior to the beginning of the activity.

- To ensure that the participant reaps the benefits of being engaged, please adapt any and all activities to the participants functional level.

Program Name: Beer and Wine Word Scramble   **Date:** _____

Leader: _____   **Time:** _____

Objective:

- Stimulate cognitive functioning
- Increase self-worth and improve self-esteem
- Increase socialization
- Foster friendship, laughter and closeness
- Provide a sense of accomplishment
- Stimulate memory
- Have some fun!

Materials:

- Flat surface for participant to write on
- Templates on the following pages provided
- Pen, pencil or high lighter

Note: If a participant is in a bed, recliner or wheelchair, consider using the R.O.S. Multi-Purpose Board Insert and the R.O.S. Legacy™ System Console available at R.O.S. Therapy Systems (www.therosstore.com) as an option for a flat surface to allow the participant the opportunity to fully engage in this activity.

Prerequisite Skills:

Every person has his or her own unique physical/cognitive abilities and needs. How a participant responds to an activity will dictate how the caregiver will modify or adapt a Lesson Plan to meet individual client needs and abilities – now and in the future.

Program Name: Beer and Wine Word Scramble   **Date:** _____

Leader: _____   **Time:** _____

Activity Outline:

Leader explains to participant that they will be working on a word scramble puzzle

1. Use the following templates to enjoy word scramble based on topics of interest

Option 1: Based on participant abilities, participant completes activity on their own

Option 2: Based on participant abilities, leader assists with finding answers

Option 3: Based on participant abilities, leader and participant have discussion based on words and topic included in this activity

Evaluation:

Red Wine Terms 1 - Word Scramble

1. NSOE

   _ _ _ _

2. PTMDNOIE

   _ _ _ _ _ _ _ _

3. VIENNTR

   _ _ _ _ _ _ _

4. BNWAYR

   _ _ _ _ _ _

5. JMAMY

   _ _ _ _ _

6. TAINSNN

   _ _ _ _ _ _ _

7. MLROET

   _ _ _ _ _ _

8. VNERYDIA

   _ _ _ _ _ _ _ _

9. BLEOTT

   _ _ _ _ _ _

10. MEILSCAUN

    _ _ _ _ _ _ _ _ _

Red Wine Terms 2 - Word Scramble

1. PMEIRERCUR _ _ _ _ _ _ _ _ _ _

2. VGENITA _ _ _ _ _ _ _

3. BERLRA _ _ _ _ _ _

4. PNITONIOR _ _ _ _ _ _ _ _ _

5. FIISHN _ _ _ _ _ _

6. CNAIITH _ _ _ _ _ _ _

7. BULHS _ _ _ _ _

8. OOOEGNLY _ _ _ _ _ _ _ _

9. CRATEL _ _ _ _ _ _

10. BGNU _ _ _ _

White Wine Terms 1 - Word Scramble

1. BLACN _ _ _ _ _

2. RYAC _ _ _ _

3. CAHPMEAGN _ _ _ _ _ _ _ _ _

4. OKA _ _ _

5. LOREI _ _ _ _ _

6. CBHAISL _ _ _ _ _ _ _

7. VAITEGN _ _ _ _ _ _ _

8. BUUOQTE _ _ _ _ _ _ _

9. RLGNSEII _ _ _ _ _ _ _ _

10. GRIOIG _ _ _ _ _ _

White Wine Terms 2 - Word Scramble

1. SIPRTRZE _ _ _ _ _ _ _ _

2. CHNIEN _ _ _ _ _ _

3. CODRNANHAY _ _ _ _ _ _ _ _ _ _

4. VSEIN _ _ _ _ _

5. ZLFENAIND _ _ _ _ _ _ _ _ _

6. FERTEENDM _ _ _ _ _ _ _ _ _

7. MOSIAM _ _ _ _ _ _

8. COROEP _ _ _ _ _ _

9. SEMEIORLM _ _ _ _ _ _ _ _ _

10. BDORUAEX _ _ _ _ _ _ _ _

Beer Terms 1 - Word Scramble

1. FEMTREN _ _ _ _ _ _ _

2. HPOS _ _ _ _

3. SEINT _ _ _ _ _

4. BWER _ _ _ _

5. FAMO _ _ _ _

6. AMREB _ _ _ _ _

7. AEL _ _ _

8. LGEAR _ _ _ _ _

9. YADR _ _ _ _

10. MGU _ _ _

Beer Terms 2 - Word Scramble

1. PBU _ _ _

2. YAETS _ _ _ _ _

3. BALRYE _ _ _ _ _ _

4. FHGTIL _ _ _ _ _ _

5. BWRRYEE _ _ _ _ _ _ _

6. KGE _ _ _

7. BLARRE _ _ _ _ _ _

8. CSKA _ _ _ _

9. PISLNRE _ _ _ _ _ _ _

10. BEOTTL _ _ _ _ _ _

Bartender Terms 1 - Word Scramble

1. BOBONUR

2. AVRHEYLNGLBAAVVRE

3. DUELMRD

4. ADNRGMRNEARI

5. EQIALTU

6. NIGARSH

7. BACAUMS

8. BETTRIS

9. TEIMLG

10. ENELDBR

Bartender Terms 3 - Word Scramble

1. ENFITRS

_ _ _ _ _ _ _

2. ITWST

_ _ _ _ _

3. BTUMRLE

_ _ _ _ _ _ _

4. WLIEZZS

_ _ _ _ _ _ _

5. OTMLOCSILN

_ _ _ _ _ _ _ _ _ _

6. IGGERJ

_ _ _ _ _ _

7. CUABIELBR

_ _ _ _ _ _ _ _ _

8. DLOESHADNOFI

_ _ _ _ _ _ _ _ _ _ _ _

9. OCRRSCEKW

_ _ _ _ _ _ _ _ _

10. USTYRIALN

_ _ _ _ _ _ _ _ _

Red Wine Terms 1 - Word Scramble

1. NSOE   N o s e

2. PTMDNOIE   P i e d m o n t

3. VIENNTR   V i n t n e r

4. BNWAYR   B r a w n y

5. JMAMY   J a m m y

6. TAINSNN   T a n n i n s

7. MLROET   M e r l o t

8. VNERYDIA   V i n e y a r d

9. BLEOTT   B o t t l e

10. MEILSCAUN   M a s c u l i n e

Red Wine Terms 2 - Word Scramble

1. PMEIRERCUR   P r e m i e r C r u

2. VGENITA   V i n t a g e

3. BERLRA   B a r r e l

4. PNITONIOR   P i n o t N o i r

5. FIISHN   F i n i s h

6. CNAIITH   C h i a n t i

7. BULHS   B l u s h

8. OOOEGNLY   O e n o l o g y

9. CRATEL   C l a r e t

10. BGNU   B u n g

White Wine Terms 1 - Word Scramble

1. BLACN   B l a n c

2. RYAC   R a c y

3. CAHPMEAGN   C h a m p a g n e

4. OKA   O a k

5. LOREI   L o i r e

6. CBHAISL   C h a b l i s

7. VAITEGN   V i n t a g e

8. BUUOQTE   B o u q u e t

9. RLGNSEII   R i e s l i n g

10. GRIOIG   G r i g i o

White Wine Terms 2 - Word Scramble

1. SIPRTRZE — S p r i t z e r

2. CHNIEN — C h e n i n

3. CODRNANHAY — C h a r d o n n a y

4. VSEIN — V i n e s

5. ZLFENAIND — Z i n f a n d e l

6. FERTEENDM — F e r m e n t e d

7. MOSIAM — M i m o s a

8. COROEP — C o o p e r

9. SEMEIORLM — S o m m e l i e r

10. BDORUAEX — B o r d e a u x

Beer Terms 1 - Word Scramble

1. FEMTREN — F e r m e n t
2. HPOS — H o p s
3. SEINT — S t e i n
4. BWER — B r e w
5. FAMO — F o a m
6. AMREB — A m b e r
7. AEL — A l e
8. LGEAR — L a g e r
9. YADR — Y a r d
10. MGU — M u g

Beer Terms 2 - Word Scramble

1. PBU — P u b

2. YAETS — Y e a s t

3. BALRYE — B a r l e y

4. FHGTIL — F l i g h t

5. BWRRYEE — B r e w e r y

6. KGE — K e g

7. BLARRE — B a r r e l

8. CSKA — C a s k

9. PISLNRE — P i l s n e r

10. BEOTTL — B o t t l e

Bartender Terms 1 - Word Scramble

1. BOBONUR — B o u r b o n

2. AVRHEYLNGLBAAWRE — H a r v e y   W a l l b a n g e r

3. DUELMRD — M u d d l e r

4. ADNRGMRNEARI — G r a n d   M a r n i e r

5. EQIALTU — T e q u i l a

6. NIGARSH — G a r n i s h

7. BACAUMS — S a m b u c a

8. BETTRIS — B i t t e r s

9. TEIMLG — G i m l e t

10. ENELDBR — B l e n d e r

Bartender Terms 3 - Word Scramble

1. ENFITRS

S n i f t e r

2. ITWST

T w i s t

3. BTUMRLE

T u m b l e r

4. WLIEZZS

S w i z z l e

5. OTMLOCSILN

T o m C o l l i n s

6. IGGERJ

J i g g e r

7. CUABIELBR

C u b a L i b r e

8. DLOESHADNOFI

O l d F a s h i o n e d

9. OCRRSCEKW

C o r k s c r e w

10. USTYRIALN

R u s t y N a i l

Activity Lesson Plans

Wine, Beer and Bartending Word Search

Wine, Beer and Bartending Word Search

- The following pages contain basic templates that can be used with anyone. The leader must allow for the participant to be successful.

- The leader should read all step-by-step directions of an Activity Outline before beginning an activity with a participant. The step-by-step directions are general guidelines for the leader/caregiver to use and potentially modify in order to help the participant successfully engage in the chosen activity.

- The leader must always be present when engaging the participant in an activity.

- The leader must take all necessary and reasonable precautions to ensure the safety of the participant.

- The leader should have necessary materials ready and prepared prior to the beginning of the activity.

- To ensure that the participant reaps the benefits of being engaged, please adapt any and all activities to the participants functional level.

Program Name: Beer and Wine Word Search   **Date:** _____

Leader: _____   **Time:** _____

Objective:

- Stimulate cognitive functioning
- Increase self-worth and improve self-esteem
- Increase socialization
- Foster friendship, laughter and closeness
- Provide a sense of accomplishment
- Stimulate memory
- Have some fun!

Materials:

- Flat surface for participant to write on
- Templates on the following pages provided
- Pen, pencil or high lighter

Note: If a participant is in a bed, recliner or wheelchair, consider using the R.O.S. Multi-Purpose Board Insert and the R.O.S. Legacy™ System Console available at R.O.S. Therapy Systems (www.therosstore.com) as an option for a flat surface to allow the participant the opportunity to fully engage in this activity.

Prerequisite Skills:

Every person has his or her own unique physical/cognitive abilities and needs. How a participant responds to an activity will dictate how the caregiver will modify or adapt a Lesson Plan to meet individual client needs and abilities – now and in the future.

Program Name: Beer and Wine Word Search   **Date:** _____

Leader: _____   **Time:** _____

Activity Outline:

The leader explains to the participant that they will be working on a Word Search puzzle.

1. Use the following templates to enjoy Word Search based on topics of interest.

Option 1: Based on the participants abilities, the participant completes the activity on their own.

Option 2: Based on the participants abilities, the leader assists with finding answers.

Option 3: Based on the participants abilities, the leader and participant have a discussion based on words and topics included in this activity.

Evaluation:

Red Wine Terms 1 - Wordsearch

Tannins

Brawny

Jammy

Masculine

Piedmont

Bottle

Nose

Vintner

Merlot

Vineyard

```
Y I U T J D J M B O T T L E N L
Y N J A Q S Z Z P H C R J N R N
J Q A P Y M K L F A M G G U W
Z G M I L E Q K R J Z I N N M L
U U M E K R M T Q V I N T N E R
D U Y D Q L Z A M X X F U H O J
A F H M S O D N H D B S V F T L
M X M O N T I N A D L S I M V Z
A P G N D H W I U G C C N V C L
S T E T Y H Z N A G U I E G U Q
C O S B T Z U S Y Z U N Y I B J
U J V O R Q C F Y J K O A E L P
L K J Z J A E U E F Y S R F I K
I Y P Y O U W I J A Q E D S G R
N P Y J J B U N Y N H U I P O B
E D H N U T Y T Y I W Z A S W A
```

Red Wine Terms 2 - Wordsearch

Y	C	Y	L	W	Z	A	S	F	Q	W	R	C	B	Y	G
M	R	I	H	C	F	I	A	X	E	A	B	U	N	G	X
Z	W	K	Y	E	Y	Q	S	T	H	G	M	M	C	F	A
V	I	N	T	A	G	E	M	R	L	U	A	W	O	F	E
S	C	Z	B	C	P	P	J	T	F	I	N	I	S	H	X
V	L	N	I	N	G	C	H	I	A	N	T	I	P	C	H
X	P	P	Z	F	N	C	L	A	R	E	T	S	R	J	X
H	T	I	M	K	Z	F	B	L	U	S	H	S	E	Y	H
T	O	N	C	G	O	E	N	O	L	O	G	Y	M	R	T
Y	H	O	U	P	O	R	Z	C	N	J	F	K	I	C	O
T	M	T	L	E	N	T	W	B	R	Z	V	H	E	O	E
G	L	N	R	W	J	B	N	R	A	P	X	X	R	G	Q
O	K	O	B	O	Q	X	H	Y	G	R	F	A	C	R	M
U	V	I	O	A	F	V	Y	X	F	A	R	E	R	E	T
T	E	R	Y	U	J	Z	P	C	D	L	U	E	U	Y	U
M	B	U	I	W	H	N	E	M	I	A	M	J	L	P	N

Pinot Noir

Oenology

Finish

Premier Cru

Blush

Chianti

Barrel

Bung

Claret

Vintage

White Wine Terms 1 - Wordsearch

Racy
Riesling
Loire
Bouquet
Blanc
Grigio
Champagne
Vintage
Oak
Chablis

C	E	B	L	Y	S	R	E	W	Y	J	P	J	E	E
Q	H	P	Y	O	T	H	I	J	U	P	E	A	O	H
O	R	A	C	E	I	J	O	E	B	U	Q	Z	Y	A
Y	B	S	B	W	G	R	X	O	S	X	P	H	Z	R
X	V	B	P	L	G	G	E	C	R	L	L	T	T	V
L	F	L	K	Q	I	R	M	V	K	M	I	M	Q	H
I	V	A	O	U	C	S	I	R	I	M	G	N	A	I
O	I	N	T	E	M	X	O	G	G	N	D	S	G	M
C	B	C	K	T	L	H	X	A	I	T	T	L	N	I
V	O	D	X	S	E	X	J	D	K	O	A	A	X	A
K	U	O	U	L	H	I	O	J	L	T	C	R	G	P
R	Q	O	M	N	R	A	Z	I	G	F	G	X	E	E
W	U	H	G	V	R	C	H	A	M	P	A	G	N	E
R	E	D	O	W	X	M	R	M	H	W	L	P	I	T
K	T	L	V	E	X	I	V	R	R	A	C	Y	U	R

White Wine Terms 2 - Wordsearch

Chenin
Chardonnay
Cooper
Sommelier
Bordeaux
Fermented
Vines
Mimosa
Spritzer
Zinfandel

```
O S B L K N V B D Y Q R B M R C R
F K A U B N F S B U D C F T J H H
X H B X D C O D T B Q I M B L A F
V M F E R M E N T E D P B R O R B
T O E K Z H H G B W Z F O Y L D O
G B H C D B H C I F M S Z N O O R
M U M S G W V I N E S Y A C M N D
J M X B S J Q K J X T Y P O T N E
U H C L S O M M E L I E R I L A A
N Z V C K Z I N F A N D E L K H Y U
J W G J X Y A D T I V W V Q U T X
C H E N I N U B N C J S B X G K W
O Z I B H Z J Q N F I Q G K K N K
O S T D I J N D K B V N Q Q H E N
P A S P R I T Z E R M I M O S A I
E I S I F B M N Y F W R G E I F L
R T A V N S T R L Y T B A W M I D
```

Beer Terms 1 - Wordsearch

H	Y	O	F	G	H	S	U	O	S	V	E	K	R
W	L	V	E	Q	Y	O	T	P	Q	D	O	M	R
R	R	G	R	O	A	N	P	L	F	Y	I	Q	R
D	Z	V	M	B	R	Z	O	S	X	R	B	G	H
A	P	J	E	T	D	Z	T	H	O	V	I	N	L
C	K	H	N	T	I	Q	J	A	G	K	W	G	J
I	B	L	T	S	C	G	J	A	L	A	U	U	R
R	R	K	N	D	E	J	H	A	Q	A	Q	O	E
F	E	O	S	T	E	I	N	A	P	Y	G	W	H
N	W	Q	G	V	E	W	W	M	X	B	X	E	E
F	J	V	Z	W	S	W	O	B	A	G	C	X	R
P	O	D	L	W	P	E	U	E	L	V	U	P	Z
A	E	A	P	G	I	K	T	R	E	D	L	M	A
W	F	J	M	M	U	G	F	T	B	M	X	P	G

Brew

Mug

Yard

Amber

Ferment

Ale

Hops

Stein

Foam

Lager

Beer Terms 2 - Wordsearch

Word list: Keg, Barrel, Pilsner, Flight, Brewery, Barley, Yeast, Bottle, Pub, Cask

B	A	R	R	E	L	V	X	B	W	K	B	Z	X	W
K	E	G	C	D	B	W	D	B	F	H	A	U	E	J
E	C	Z	M	T	R	F	K	O	Z	F	R	G	W	A
T	W	N	L	F	E	N	Z	T	I	B	L	E	D	K
J	L	K	R	H	W	O	U	T	H	E	C	Y	P	
X	K	C	T	V	E	P	F	L	A	P	Y	A	E	K
Q	M	G	P	J	R	G	Y	E	L	O	B	S	A	R
K	L	L	U	H	Y	B	J	T	K	V	S	K	S	R
S	X	N	B	F	T	X	A	J	H	L	Q	C	T	X
N	R	W	O	F	E	Q	Z	U	Z	M	V	Q	G	R
K	M	E	T	L	F	E	O	W	B	S	D	K	U	Y
W	L	J	E	P	A	A	B	I	O	V	D	A	P	
P	I	L	S	N	E	R	K	F	L	I	G	H	T	J
A	E	Z	G	E	A	U	T	Z	G	N	B	Y	I	T
Y	X	Y	N	R	I	F	O	Q	R	D	L	T	C	R

Bartender Terms 1 - Crossword

Gimlet

Harvey Wallbanger

Muddler

Garnish

Blender

Grand Marnier

Bitters

Sambuca

Tequila

Bourbon

```
L G R A N D M A R N I E R I P N P Z
B X H Z R Z X H V P R S Z H M X U W
Y N Z I J K B A K I H S M J I B Q A
Q M T X L P N Y D C A T R Q Z Z C O
I S H G L Q H P U R S O B I X D O
G A J B O U R B O N V M A H Q H N R
P W R C A U T U T M E F V M E G H N
A R H U M I E B N T Y T Q R B Y A R
T W O G G M Q A K J W R J O G U Q A
W H Y P I U U B M Y A E M D A R C H
U W Y E M D I N T O L K F G R S L A
P B E D L D L U U M L B L E N D E R
J X Y Z E L A U I A B V J Z I L Y G
Y L N N T E V U Z W A E T W S K G P
L I U Q L R R L U M N Z Z Y H S V I
G G V A R Z T D K Q G A P Q C S S O
Y E B I T T E R S T E K B H Y B B F
N F O X H F L P Y Z R Z D K N I F J
```

Bartender Terms 3 - Wordsearch

Word List:

- Rusty Nail
- Old Fashioned
- Tom Collins
- Cuba Libre
- Swizzle
- Corkscrew
- Tumbler
- Snifter
- Jigger
- Twist

E	R	U	F	S	B	U	I	H	T	C	O	H	U	T	G	G	G
L	Y	H	G	U	K	O	X	Z	G	U	U	A	F	I	T	M	B
O	B	E	P	N	W	D	R	Z	U	M	B	R	O	F	C	T	I
V	Q	N	U	G	C	F	I	D	Y	B	A	U	U	K	R	F	N
D	O	G	I	K	I	O	N	Y	L	L	D	V	U	M	H	F	Z
S	Y	C	T	V	Q	E	R	P	G	E	I	T	W	I	S	T	Z
W	R	V	C	P	R	H	J	K	E	R	B	C	H	E	C	C	P
I	J	I	G	G	E	R	L	R	S	R	R	U	W	L	E	Y	Y
N	F	Z	J	T	W	P	J	D	U	C	E	N	V	H	Y	D	I
Z	B	A	I	C	H	F	J	X	S	S	R	J	D	T	V	W	L
L	P	R	D	K	D	V	Q	N	S	T	E	A	O	R	W	M	L
E	K	Q	C	W	A	Q	O	N	I	D	C	Y	W	T	T	E	Y
P	V	I	O	V	Q	R	Q	N	F	O	K	Z	N	H	G	O	P
R	X	B	A	Z	W	J	N	Y	T	W	P	W	Y	A	B	F	I
Q	O	W	R	J	X	B	Q	S	E	C	E	A	G	W	I	W	F
J	K	R	I	D	W	R	L	X	R	F	W	Y	H	N	T	L	K
J	Q	X	B	K	O	L	D	F	A	S	H	I	O	N	E	D	S
T	O	M	C	O	L	L	I	N	S	X	O	S	R	Y	Y	H	C

Red Wine Terms 1 - Wordsearch

Tannins

Brawny

Jammy

Masculine

Piedmont

Bottle

Nose

Vintner

Merlot

Vineyard

Red Wine Terms 2 - Wordsearch

Pinot Noir

Oenology

Finish

Premier Cru

Blush

Chianti

Barrel

Bung

Claret

Vintage

Y	C	Y	L	W	Z	A	S	F	Q	W	R	C	B	Y	G
M	R	I	H	C	F	I	A	X	E	A	B	U	N	G	X
Z	W	K	Y	E	Y	Q	S	T	H	G	M	M	C	F	A
V	I	N	T	A	G	E	M	R	L	U	A	W	O	F	E
S	C	Z	B	C	P	P	J	T	F	I	N	I	S	H	X
V	L	I	N	G	C	H	I	A	N	T	I	P	C	H	
X	P	Z	F	N	C	L	A	R	E	T	S	R	J	X	
H	T	O	M	K	Z	F	B	L	U	S	H	S	E	Y	H
T	O	Y	H	C	G	O	E	N	O	L	O	G	Y	M	R	T
T	M	T	L	E	N	T	W	B	R	Z	V	H	E	O	E
G	L	N	R	W	J	B	N	R	A	P	X	X	R	G	Q
O	K	O	B	O	Q	X	H	Y	G	R	F	A	C	R	M
U	V	I	O	A	F	V	Y	X	F	A	R	E	R	E	T
T	E	R	Y	U	J	Z	P	C	D	L	U	E	U	Y	U
M	B	U	I	W	H	N	E	M	I	A	M	J	L	P	N

61

White Wine Terms 1 - Wordsearch

Racy
Riesling
Loire
Bouquet
Blanc
Grigio
Champagne
Vintage
Oak
Chablis

White Wine Terms 2 - Wordsearch

Chenin

Chardonnay

Cooper

Sommelier

Bordeaux

Fermented

Vines

Mimosa

Spritzer

Zinfandel

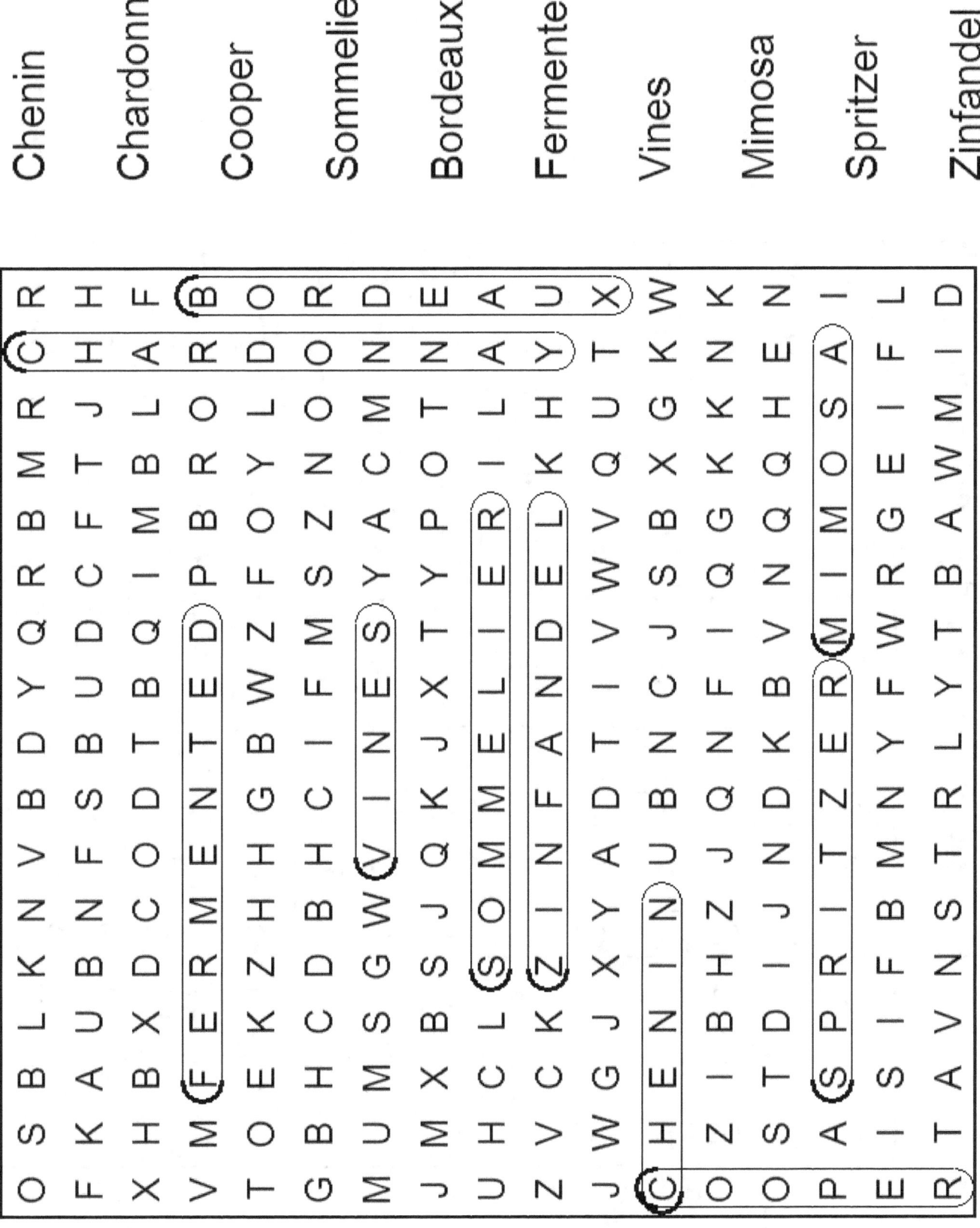

Beer Terms 1 - Wordsearch

Brew

Mug

Yard

Amber

Ferment

Ale

Hops

Stein

Foam

Lager

Beer Terms 2 - Wordsearch

Keg
Barrel
Pilsner
Flight
Brewery
Barley
Yeast
Bottle
Pub
Cask

B	V	B	K	L	F	Y	W	Z	X	W
K	X	A	H	R	K	C	U	E	X	J
E	B	H	F	H	Z	G	E	W	G	A
E	W	D	B	N	O	R	B	L	E	K
T	D	R	F	Z	U	I	H	E	D	K
W	K	O	N	F	T	B	L	A	Y	P
N	C	T	E	H	R	L	H	E	C	K
L	T	E	W	O	V	A	O	A	A	R
K	V	L	U	P	E	P	U	S	S	R
C	K	T	P	F	R	L	T	K	C	X
G	C	B	J	G	J	O	V	S	Q	R
M	G	F	U	R	H	B	H	Z	G	Y
L	L	E	B	Y	Y	X	J	U	D	D
N	X	Q	X	B	T	A	M	Z	K	K
R	N	Z	O	T	J	Q	V	U	V	A
W	R	U	W	F	H	U	Q	M	Z	D
O	W	Z	B	E	A	L	V	O	U	P
F	K	U	S	Q	J	F	Q	B	D	A
E	M	M	D	U	H	E	F	W	K	R
T	E	B	K	Z	A	O	E	B	U	A
L	T	S	U	N	B	Z	A	S	Y	B
U	L	D	P	R	I	P	A	D	D	I
J	U	K	A	Y	O	A	R	B	A	O
E	J	U	B	R	J	A	I	I	P	A
P	E	K	F	L	U	R	O	O	D	R
I	A	Z	G	E	A	U	T	Z	G	N
L	Z	X	Y	N	R	I	F	O	Q	R
S	G	Y	N	R	I	F	O	Q	R	D
N	E	A	U	T	Z	G	N	B	Y	I
E	R	K	F	L	I	G	H	T	J	T

Bartender Terms 1 - Crossword

- Gimlet
- Harvey Wallbanger
- Muddler
- Garnish
- Blender
- Grand Marnier
- Bitters
- Sambuca
- Tequila
- Bourbon

Bartender Terms 3 - Wordsearch

Rusty Nail

Old Fashioned

Tom Collins

Cuba Libre

Swizzle

Corkscrew

Tumbler

Snifter

Jigger

Twist

Activity Lesson Plans

Wine, Beer and Bartending Crossword

Wine, Beer and Bartending Crossword

- The following pages contain basic templates that can be used with anyone. The leader must allow for the participant to be successful.

- The leader should read all step-by-step directions of an Activity Outline before beginning an activity with a participant. The step-by-step directions are general guidelines for the leader/caregiver to use and potentially modify in order to help the participant successfully engage in the chosen activity.

- The leader must always be present when engaging the participant in an activity.

- The leader must take all necessary and reasonable precautions to ensure the safety of the participant.

- The leader should have necessary materials ready and prepared prior to the beginning of the activity.

- To ensure that the participant reaps the benefits of being engaged, please adapt any and all activities to the participants functional level.

Program Name: Beer and Wine Crossword   **Date:** _____

Leader: _____   **Time:** _____

Objective:

- Stimulate cognitive functioning
- Increase self-worth and improve self-esteem
- Increase socialization
- Foster friendship, laughter and closeness
- Provide a sense of accomplishment
- Stimulate memory
- Have some fun!

Materials:

- Flat surface for participant to write on
- Templates on the following pages provided
- Pen, pencil or high lighter

Note: If a participant is in a bed, recliner or wheelchair, consider using the R.O.S. Multi-Purpose Board Insert and the R.O.S. Legacy™ System Console available at R.O.S. Therapy Systems (www.therosstore.com) as an option for a flat surface to allow the participant the opportunity to fully engage in this activity.

Prerequisite Skills:

Every person has his or her own unique physical/cognitive abilities and needs. How a participant responds to an activity will dictate how the caregiver will modify or adapt a Lesson Plan to meet individual client needs and abilities – now and in the future.

Program Name: Beer and Wine Crossword   **Date:** _____

Leader: _____   **Time:** _____

Activity Outline:

The leader explains to the participant that they will be working on a Crossword puzzle.

1. Use the following templates to enjoy a Crossword based on topics of interest.

Option 1: Based on the participants abilities, the participant completes an activity on their own.

Option 2: Based on the participants abilities, the leader assists with finding answers.

Option 3: Based on the participants abilities, the leader and the participant have a discussion based on words and topics included in this activity.

Evaluation:

Red Wine Terms 1 - Crossword

Across

3. Gives reds their bite

5. Describes reds with strong berry flavors

8. Corked wine container

9. Wine producer or seller

10. Grapes grow here

Down

1. A young red wine with harsh tannins

2. Italian region known for lusty reds

4. Describes a full-bodied, complex red wine

6. Wine's aroma

7. Bordeaux blending grape

Red Wine Terms 2 - Crossword

Across

2. The lingering taste of wine
5. English term for red Bordeaux wines
6. Pink wine made from red grapes
7. Plug used to seal a wine barrel
8. French for "first growth"

Down

1. Year grapes were harvested
3. Study of wine and wine making
4. Great red grape of Burgundy
5. Area of Tuscany known for fruity reds
7. Oak container for fermenting wine

White Wine Terms 1 - Crossword

Across

2. White wine from Burgundy
3. Wine's aroma
6. Pinot _____
7. French wine region
10. Bubbly white for toasting

Down

1. The year of harvest
4. German white wine grape
5. "White" in French
8. An acidic young white wine
9. Wood used in winemaking

White Wine Terms 2 - Crossword

Across

2. Champagne with orange juice
6. Maker of wine barrels and casks
8. Soured, as grapes
9. Grapes grow on them

Down

1. Blush-colored white
3. _____ Blanc
4. SW French wine region
5. Wine and soda drink
6. A dry white wine
7. Wine list expert

Beer Terms 1 - Crossword

Across

1. Beer grain
3. Beer head
5. Yeast's role in brewing
7. Hearty brew
9. Make beer
10. Very tall beer glass

Down

2. Decorated mug
4. Kind of beer
6. Beer glass with a handle
8. One color of beer

Beer Terms 2 - Crossword

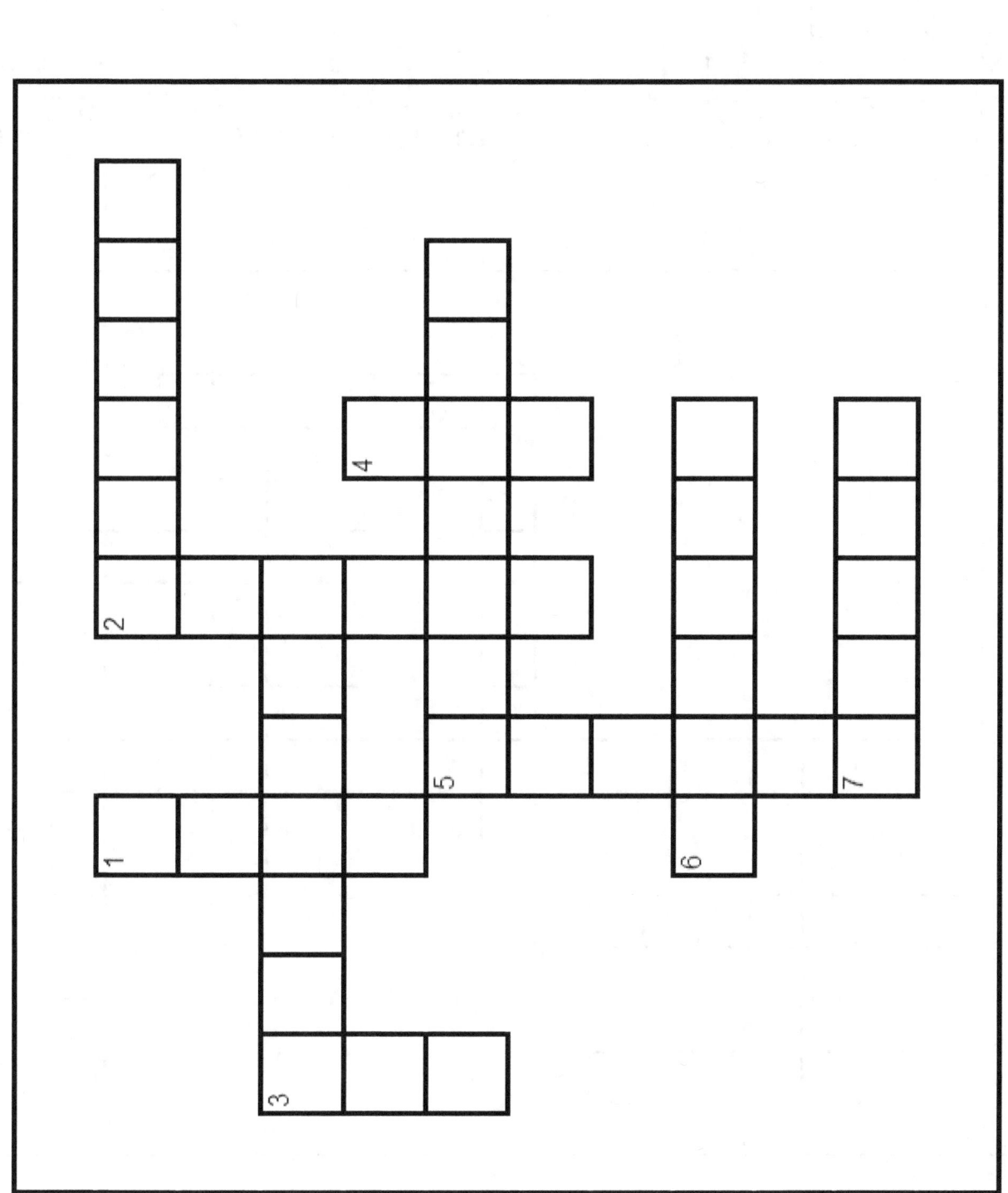

Across

2. Can alternative
3. Pale lager
5. Where beer is made
6. Beer sampler
7. Fermenting agent

Down

1. Big barrel for beer
2. "Beer _____ Polka"
3. Place to get a beer
4. Large vessel for beer
5. Beer grain

Bartender Terms 1 - Crossword

Across

4. Spirit made from agave sap
5. Italian liqueur served with coffee beans
9. Popular orange-flavored liqueur
10. Used for mashing sugar and fruit

Down

1. Compari, Unicum or Angostura
2. Kentucky's whiskey
3. Essentially a screwdriver with Galliano
6. Used to mix frozen drinks
7. Cocktail made with gin and lime juice
8. Dresses up a cocktail

Bartender Terms 3 - Crossword

Across

3. What you might do with a strip of lemon rind
4. Two-ounce measuring cup
5. A gin fizz with less fizz and no shaking
7. Half Scotch, half Drambuie
8. Stick used for stirring a cocktail
9. Rum, cola and lime

Down

1. Glassware for brandy
2. Essential for opening a bottle of wine
3. Old-fashioned or rocks glass
6. Classic whiskey cocktail garnished with orange, lemon and a cherry

White Wine Terms 1 - Crossword

Across

2. White wine from Burgundy
3. Wine's aroma
6. Pinot _____
7. French wine region
10. Bubbly white for toasting

Down

1. The year of harvest
4. German white wine grape
5. "White" in French
8. An acidic young white wine
9. Wood used in winemaking

White Wine Terms 2 - Crossword

Across

2. Champagne with orange juice
6. Maker of wine barrels and casks
8. Soured, as grapes
9. Grapes grow on them

Down

1. Blush-colored white
3. _____ Blanc
4. SW French wine region
5. Wine and soda drink
6. A dry white wine
7. Wine list expert

81

Red Wine Terms 1 - Crossword

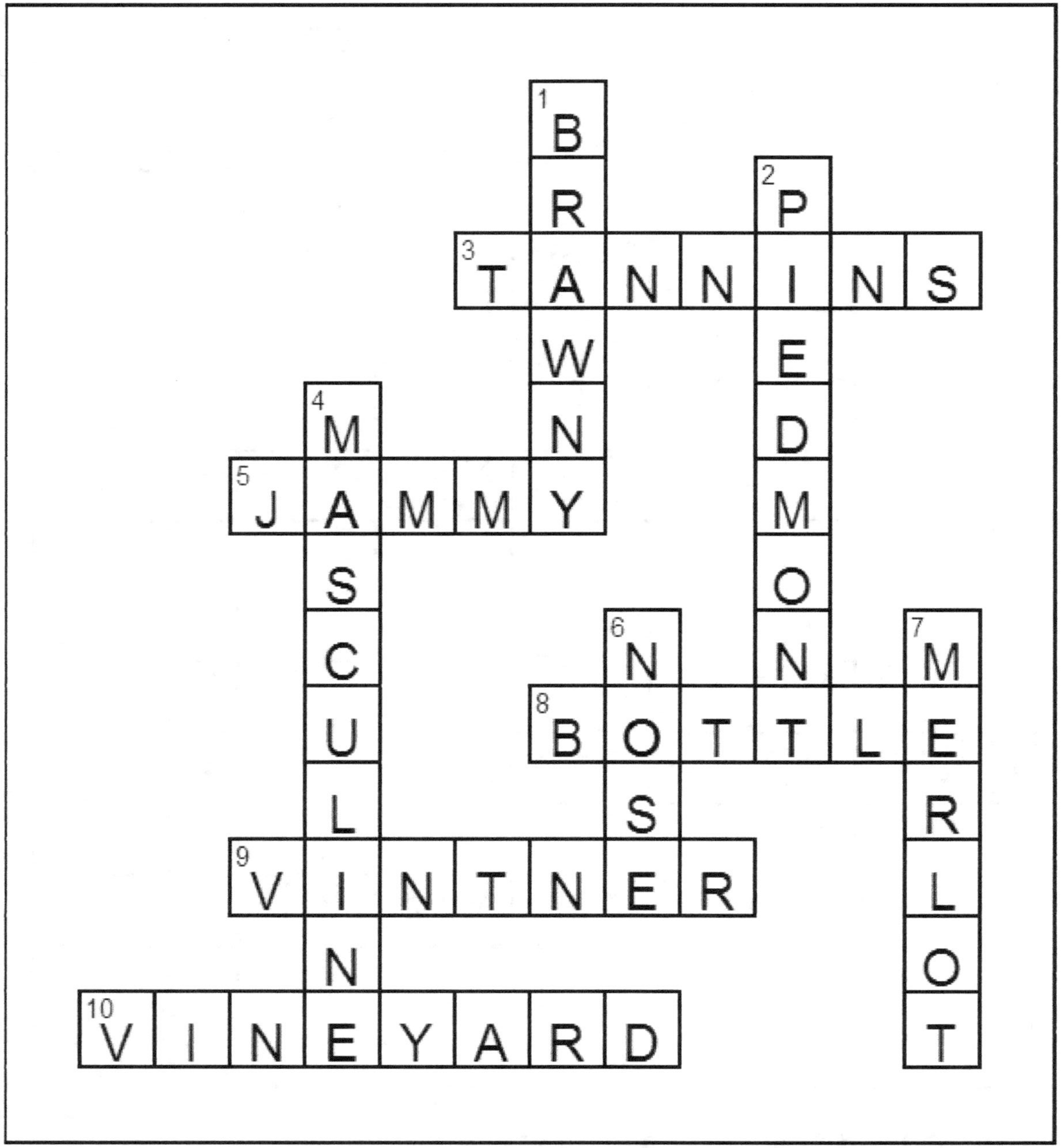
TANNINS
JAMMY
BOTTLE
VINTNER
VINEYARD
BRAWNY
PIEDMONT
MASCULINE
NOSE
MERLOT

Across

3. Gives reds their bite
5. Describes reds with strong berry flavors
8. Corked wine container
9. Wine producer or seller
10. Grapes grow here

Down

1. A young red wine with harsh tannins
2. Italian region known for lusty reds
4. Describes a full-bodied, complex red wine
6. Wine's aroma
7. Bordeaux blending grape

Red Wine Terms 2 - Crossword

Across

2. The lingering taste of wine
5. English term for red Bordeaux wines
6. Pink wine made from red grapes
7. Plug used to seal a wine barrel
8. French for "first growth"

Down

1. Year grapes were harvested
3. Study of wine and wine making
4. Great red grape of Burgundy
5. Area of Tuscany known for fruity reds
7. Oak container for fermenting wine

Beer Terms 1 - Crossword

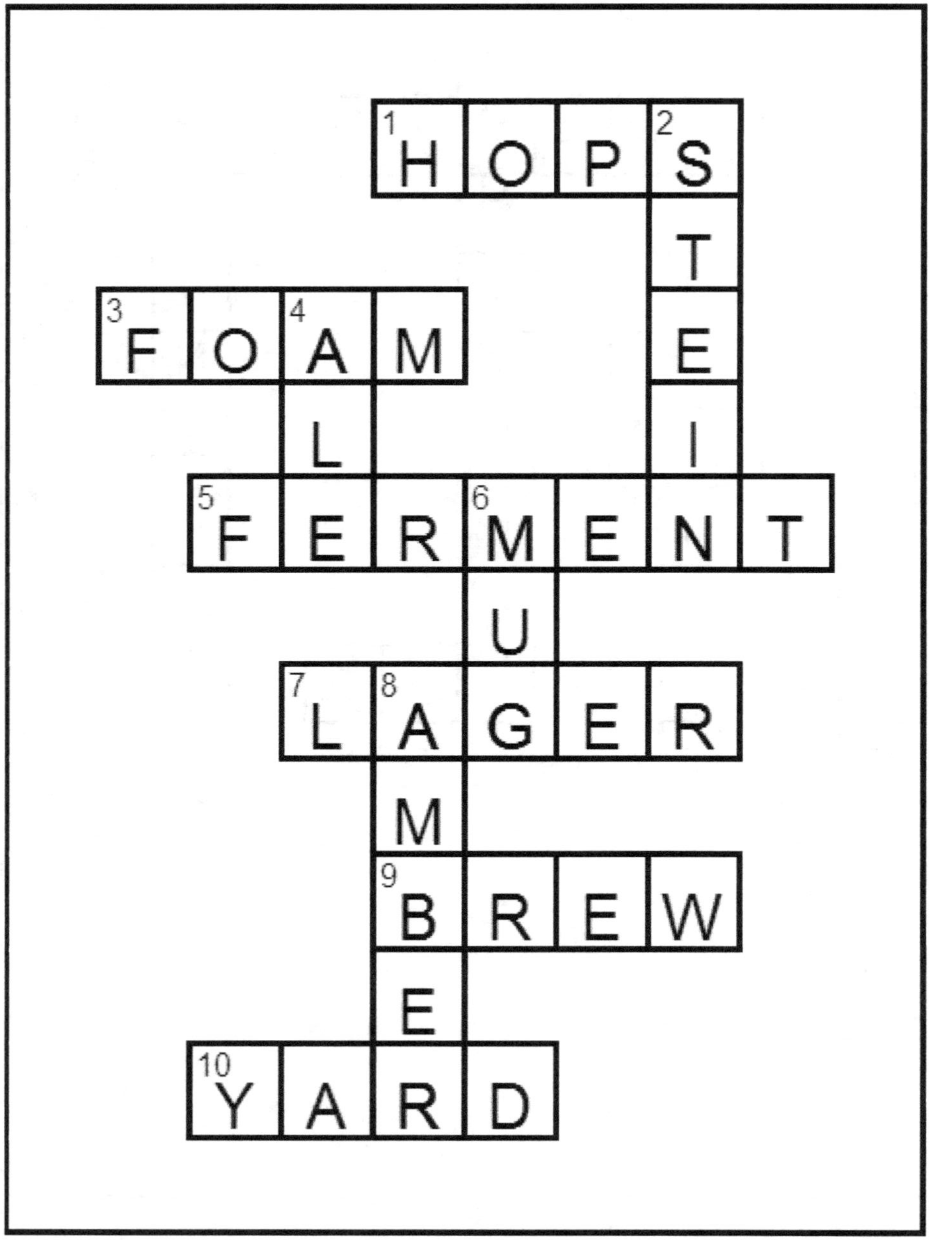
1 HOPS
2 STEIN
3 FOAM
4 ALE
5 FERMENT
6 MUG
7 LAGER
8 AMBER
9 BREW
10 YARD

Across

1. Beer grain
3. Beer head
5. Yeast's role in brewing
7. Hearty brew
9. Make beer
10. Very tall beer glass

Down

2. Decorated mug
4. Kind of beer
6. Beer glass with a handle
8. One color of beer

Beer Terms 2 - Crossword

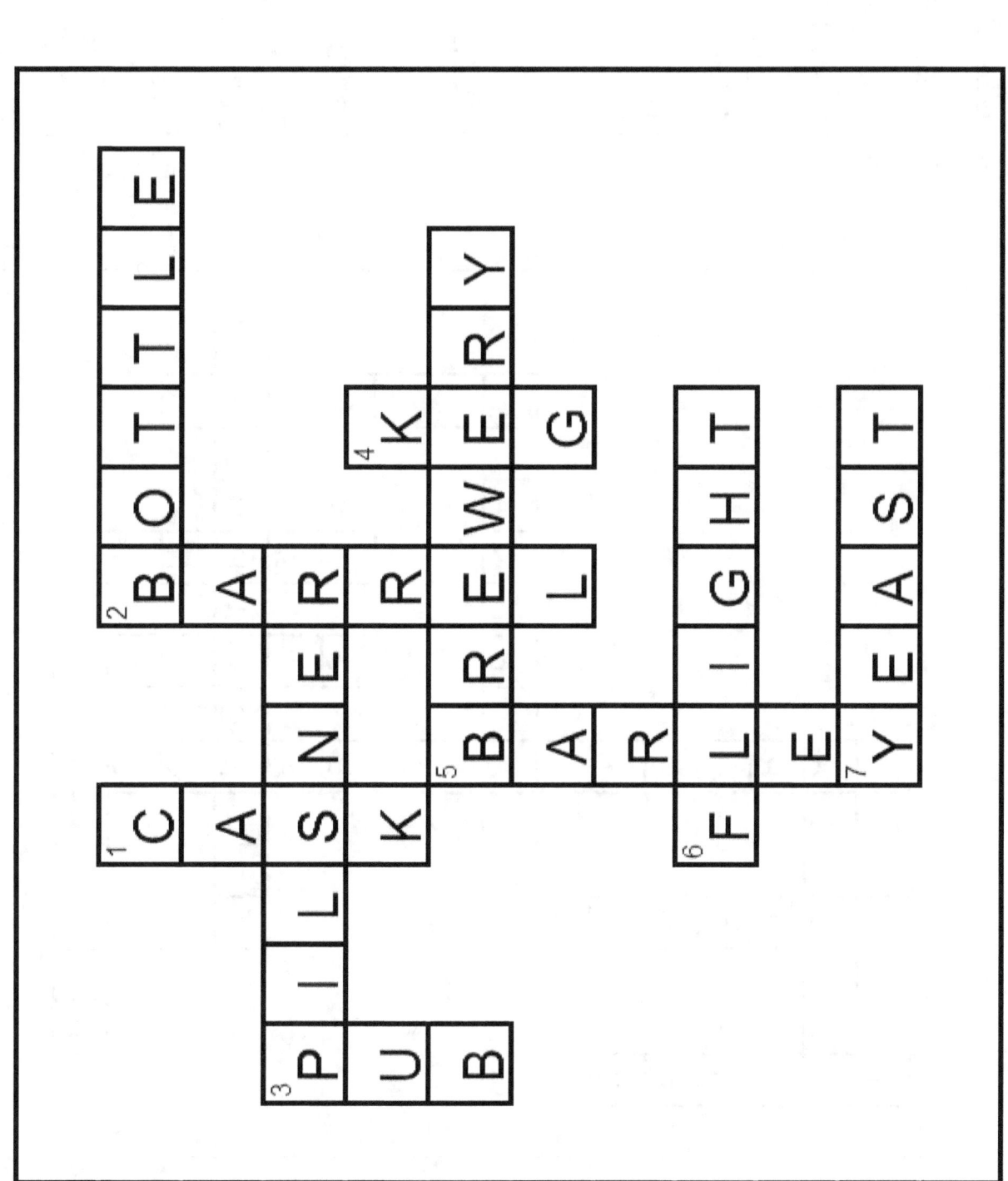

Across

2. Can alternative
3. Pale lager
5. Where beer is made
6. Beer sampler
7. Fermenting agent

Down

1. Big barrel for beer
2. "Beer _____ Polka"
3. Place to get a beer
4. Large vessel for beer
5. Beer grain

Bartender Terms 1 - Crossword

Across

4. Spirit made from agave sap
5. Italian liqueur served with coffee beans
9. Popular orange-flavored liqueur
10. Used for mashing sugar and fruit

Down

1. Compari, Unicum or Angostura
2. Kentucky's whiskey
3. Essentially a screwdriver with Galliano
6. Used to mix frozen drinks
7. Cocktail made with gin and lime juice
8. Dresses up a cocktail

Bartender Terms 3 - Crossword

Across

3. What you might do with a strip of lemon rind
4. Two-ounce measuring cup
5. A gin fizz with less fizz and no shaking
7. Half Scotch, half Drambuie
8. Stick used for stirring a cocktail
9. Rum, cola and lime

Down

1. Glassware for brandy
2. Essential for opening a bottle of wine
3. Old-fashioned or rocks glass
6. Classic whiskey cocktail garnished with orange, lemon and a cherry

Activity Lesson Plans

Wine, Beer and Bartending Code Breakers

Wine, Beer and Bartending Code Breakers

- The following pages contain basic templates that can be used with lower functioning participants. The leader must allow for the participant to be successful.

- The leader should read all step-by-step directions of an Activity Outline before beginning an activity with a participant. The step-by-step directions are general guidelines for the leader / caregiver to use and potentially modify in order to help the participant successfully engage in the chosen activity.

- The leader must always be present when engaging the participant in an activity.

- The leader must take all necessary and reasonable precautions to ensure the safety of the participant.

- The leader should have necessary materials ready and prepared prior to the beginning of the activity.

- To ensure that the participant reaps the benefits of being engaged, please adapt any and all activities to the participants functional level.

Program Name: Beer and Wine Code Breakers   **Date:** _____

Leader: _____   **Time:** _____

Objective:

- Stimulate cognitive functioning
- Increase self-worth and improve self-esteem
- Increase socialization
- Foster friendship, laughter and closeness
- Provide a sense of accomplishment
- Stimulate memory
- Have some fun!

Materials:

- Flat surface for participant to write on
- Templates on the following pages provided
- Pen, pencil or high lighter

Note: If a participant is in a bed, recliner or wheelchair, consider using the R.O.S. Multi-Purpose Board Insert and the R.O.S. Legacy™ System Console available at R.O.S. Therapy Systems (www.therosstore.com) as an option for a flat surface to allow the participant the opportunity to fully engage in this activity.

Prerequisite Skills:

Every person has his or her own unique physical/cognitive abilities and needs. How a participant responds to an activity will dictate how the caregiver will modify or adapt a Lesson Plan to meet individual client needs and abilities – now and in the future.

Program Name: Beer and Wine Code Breakers   **Date:** _____

Leader: _____   **Time:** _____

Activity Outline:

The leader explains to the participant that they will be working on Code Breaker puzzles.

1. Use the following templates to enjoy code breaker puzzles based on topics of interest.

Option 1: Based on the participants abilities, the participant completes an activity on their own.

Option 2: Based on the participants abilities, the leader assists with finding answers.

Option 3: Based on the participant abilities, the leader and the participant have a discussion based on words and topics included in this activity.

Evaluation:

Code Breakers

Use the telephone dial pad and place the correct letter above each number to break the code and solve the

Secrets of Wine Tasting

#1   Word describing a red wine high in tannins
and having a thick and soft taste

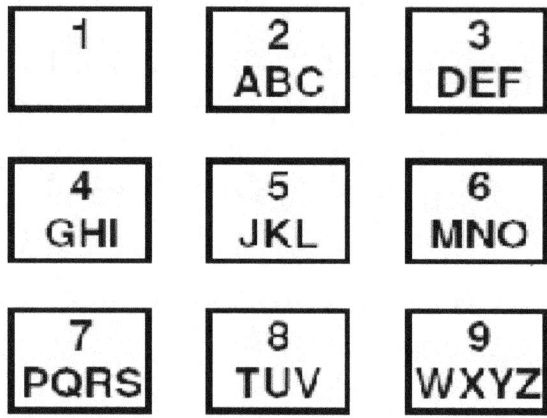

$$\frac{L}{5} \ \frac{}{3} \ \frac{}{2} \ \frac{}{8} \ \frac{}{4} \ \frac{}{3} \ \frac{}{7} \ \frac{}{9}$$

#2   Word describing a red wine that might have been
made with grapes that were overly ripe

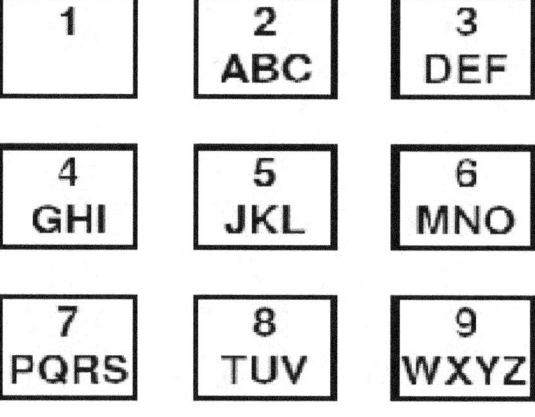

$$\frac{R}{7} \ \frac{}{2} \ \frac{}{4} \ \frac{}{7} \ \frac{}{4} \ \frac{}{6} \ \frac{}{9}$$

Code Breakers

Use the telephone dial pad and place the correct letter above each number to break the code and solve the

Secrets of Wine Tasting

#3   The puckery feeling in your mouth from drinking an especially tannic red wine

1	2 ABC	3 DEF
4 GHI	5 JKL	6 MNO
7 PQRS	8 TUV	9 WXYZ

A _ _ _ _ _ _ _ _ _
2 7 8 7 4 6 4 3 6 8

#4   A wine that is full bodied, intense and vigorous might be described as this.

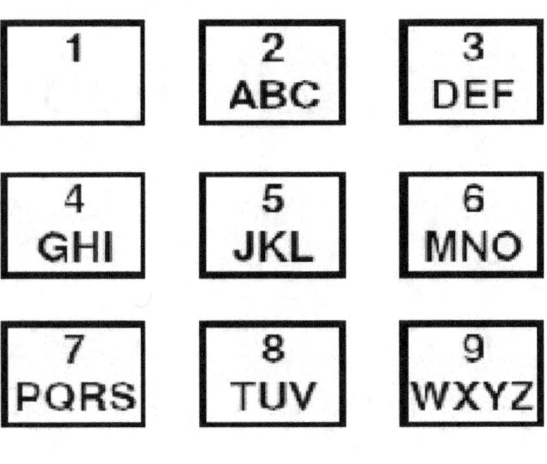

1	2 ABC	3 DEF
4 GHI	5 JKL	6 MNO
7 PQRS	8 TUV	9 WXYZ

R _ _ _ _ _
7 6 2 8 7 8

Code Breakers

Use the telephone dial pad and place the correct letter above each number to break the code and solve the

Secrets of Wine Tasting

#5   This is how you might describe a
red wine with a smooth, silky texture.

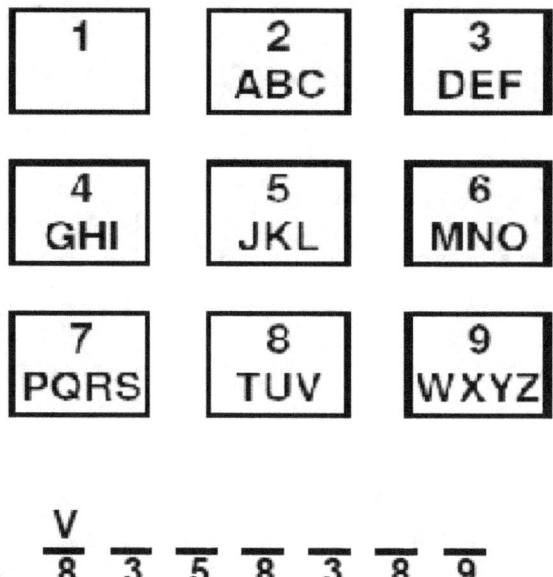

$$\frac{V}{8} \ \frac{}{3} \ \frac{}{5} \ \frac{}{8} \ \frac{}{3} \ \frac{}{8} \ \frac{}{9}$$

#6   A Burgundy with flavors of earth, undergrowth,
and decay might be described as having this taste.

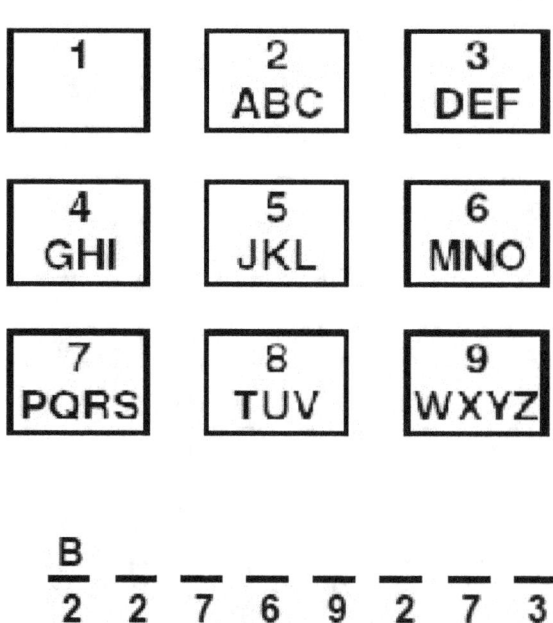

$$\frac{B}{2} \ \frac{}{2} \ \frac{}{7} \ \frac{}{6} \ \frac{}{9} \ \frac{}{2} \ \frac{}{7} \ \frac{}{3}$$

Code Breakers

Use the telephone dial pad and place the correct letter above each number to break the code and solve the

Quotations Puzzler

#1   "Beer is made by men, wine by God."

1	**2** ABC	**3** DEF
4 GHI	**5** JKL	**6** MNO
7 PQRS	**8** TUV	**9** WXYZ

M   __   __   __   __   __   __   __   __   __   __
6   2   7   8   4   6   5   8   8   4   3   7

#2   "Wine is the most healthful and
most hygienic of beverages."

1	**2** ABC	**3** DEF
4 GHI	**5** JKL	**6** MNO
7 PQRS	**8** TUV	**9** WXYZ

L   __   __   __   __   __   __   __   __   __   __   __
5   6   8   4   7   7   2   7   8   3   8   7

Code Breakers

Use the telephone dial pad and place the correct letter above each number to break the code and solve the

Quotations Puzzler

#3   "I always knew that food and wine were vital, with my mother being Italian and a good cook."

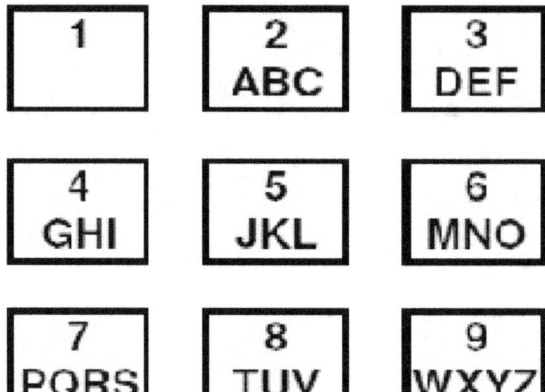

R
—
7   6   2   3   7   8   6   6   6   3   2   8   4

#4   "Quickly, bring me a beaker of wine so that I may wet my mind and say something clever."

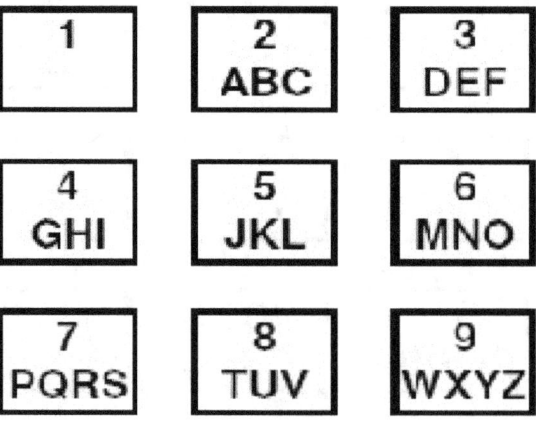

A
—
2   7   4   7   8   6   7   4   2   6   3   7

Code Breakers

Use the telephone dial pad and place the correct letter above each number to break the code and solve the

Quotations Puzzler

#5

"I cook with wine; sometimes I
even add it to the food."

1	2 ABC	3 DEF
4 GHI	5 JKL	6 MNO
7 PQRS	8 TUV	9 WXYZ

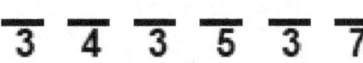

W .   _   .
—   —   — — — — — —
9   2   3 4 3 5 3 7

#6

"[A] heavy tax on wines…is a tax
on the health of our citizens."

1	2 ABC	3 DEF
4 GHI	5 JKL	6 MNO
7 PQRS	8 TUV	9 WXYZ

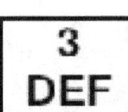

T
— — — — — —   — — — — — — — — —
8 4 6 6 2 7   5 3 3 3 3 7 7 6 6

Code Breakers - Answers
Secrets of Wine Tasting

#1   L E A T H E R Y

#2   R A I S I N Y

#3   A S T R I N G E N T

#4   R O B U S T

#5   V E L V E T Y

#6   B A R N Y A R D

Code Breakers - Answers
Quotations Puzzler

#1 M A R T I N   L U T H E R

#2 L O U I S   P A S T E U R

#3 R O B E R T   M O N D A V I

#4 A R I S T O P H A N E S

#5 W.C. F I E L D S

#6 T H O M A S   J E F F E R S O N

Code Breakers

Use the telephone dial pad and place the correct letter above each number to break the code and solve the

Beer Lovers' Puzzler

#1   Who said,"Beer is proof that God loves us?"

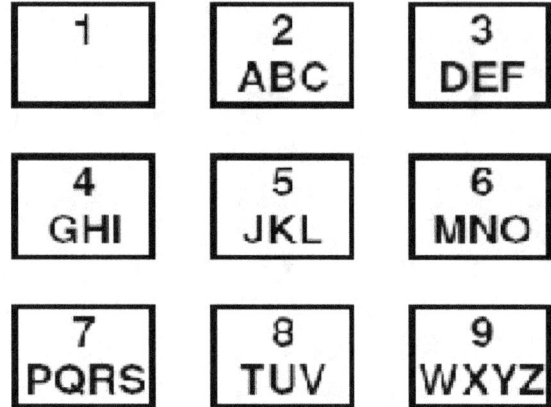

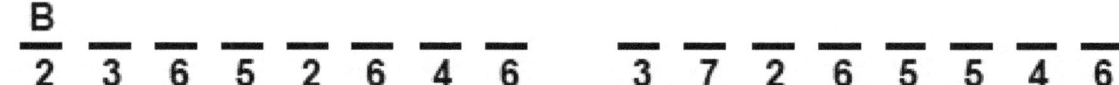

B
― ― ― ― ― ― ― ―   ― ― ― ― ― ― ―
2 3 6 5 2 6 4 6   3 7 2 6 5 5 4 6

#2   Getting home from work, this cantankerous television
character would yell, "Hey, Edith, bring me a beer!"

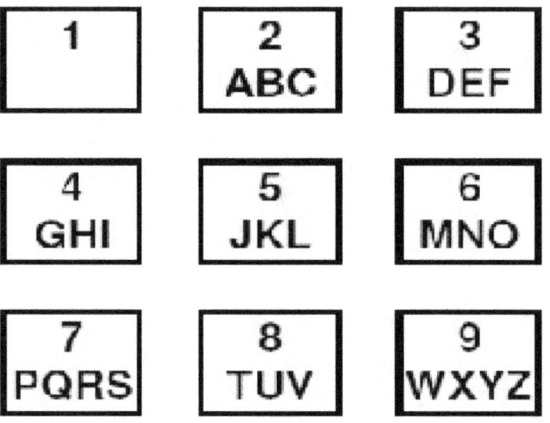

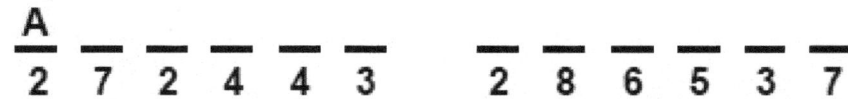

A
― ― ― ― ― ―   ― ― ― ― ― ―
2 7 2 4 4 3   2 8 6 5 3 7

Code Breakers

Use the telephone dial pad and place the correct letter above each number to break the code and solve the

Beer Lovers' Puzzler

#3   On the television show *The Simpsons*,
what is Homer Simpson's beer of choice?

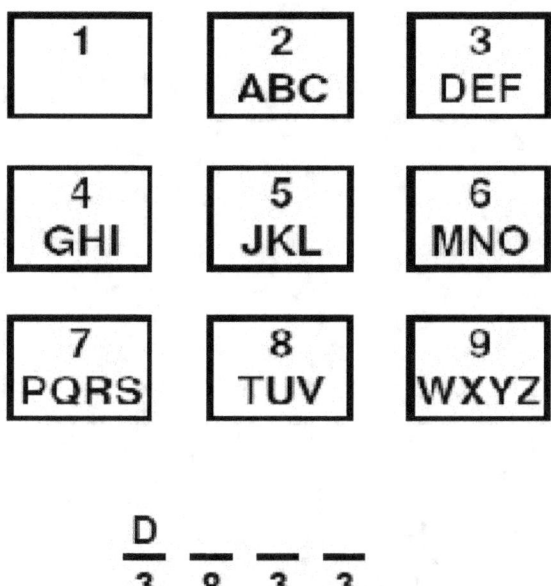

$$\frac{D}{3} \ \frac{}{8} \ \frac{}{3} \ \frac{}{3}$$

#4   In *Smokey and the Bandit*, Burt Reynolds hauled 400
cases of which brand of beer from Texas to Georgia?

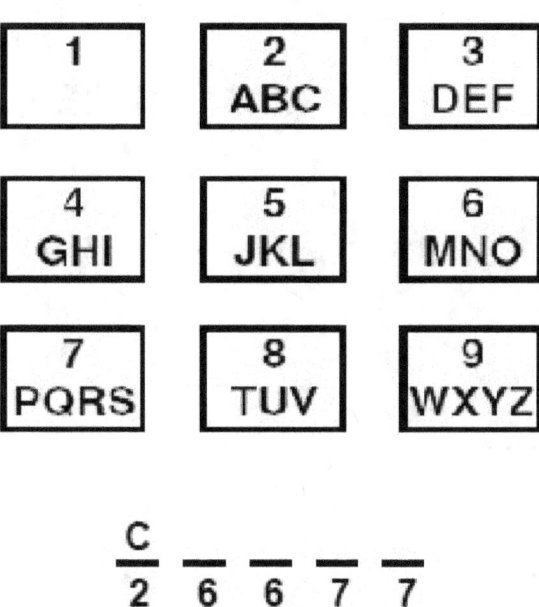

$$\frac{C}{2} \ \frac{}{6} \ \frac{}{6} \ \frac{}{7} \ \frac{}{7}$$

Code Breakers

Use the telephone dial pad and place the correct letter above each number to break the code and solve the

Beer Lovers' Puzzler

#5   What was the name of the brewery where
television's Laverne and Shirley worked?

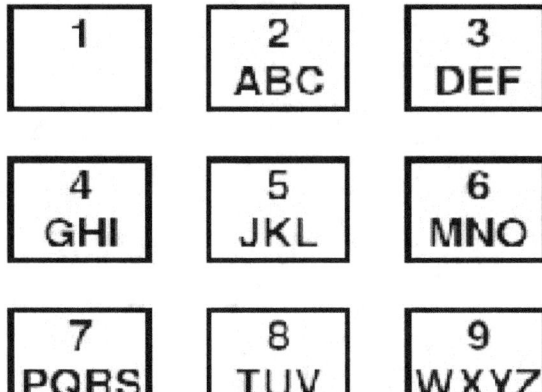

$$\frac{S}{7} \; \frac{}{4} \; \frac{}{6} \; \frac{}{8} \; \frac{}{9}$$

#6   Who were the original beer-drinking buddies
on the television comedy *Cheers?*

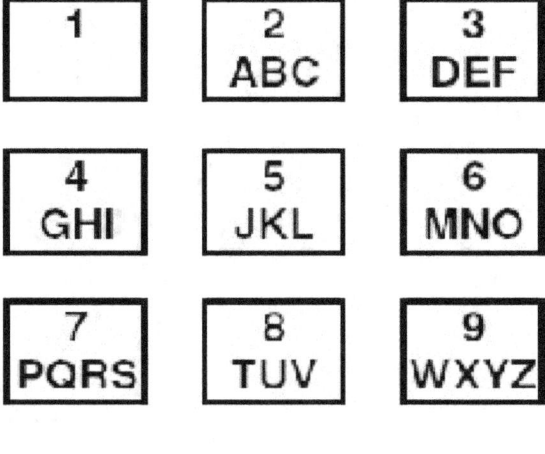

N _ _ _   A N D   _ _ _ _ _
6 6 7 6   2 5 4 3 3

Code Breakers

Use the telephone dial pad and place the correct letter above each number to break the code and solve the

Beer Slogans Boggler

#1   "Great taste, less filling"

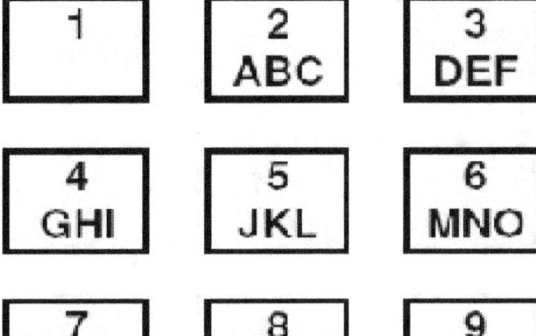

$$\frac{M}{6}\ \frac{}{4}\ \frac{}{5}\ \frac{}{5}\ \frac{}{3}\ \frac{}{7}\ \ \ \ \frac{}{5}\ \frac{}{4}\ \frac{}{4}\ \frac{}{4}\ \frac{}{8}$$

#2   "A better beer deserves a better can."

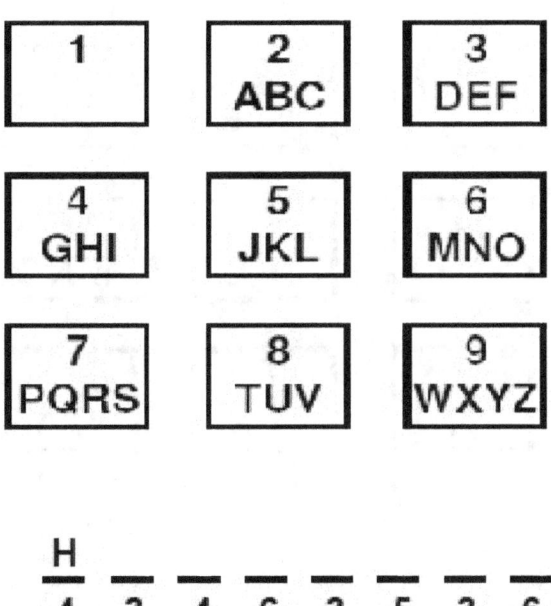

$$\frac{H}{4}\ \frac{}{3}\ \frac{}{4}\ \frac{}{6}\ \frac{}{3}\ \frac{}{5}\ \frac{}{3}\ \frac{}{6}$$

Code Breakers

Use the telephone dial pad and place the correct letter above each number to break the code and solve the

Beer Slogans Boggler

#3   The "Champagne of Beers"

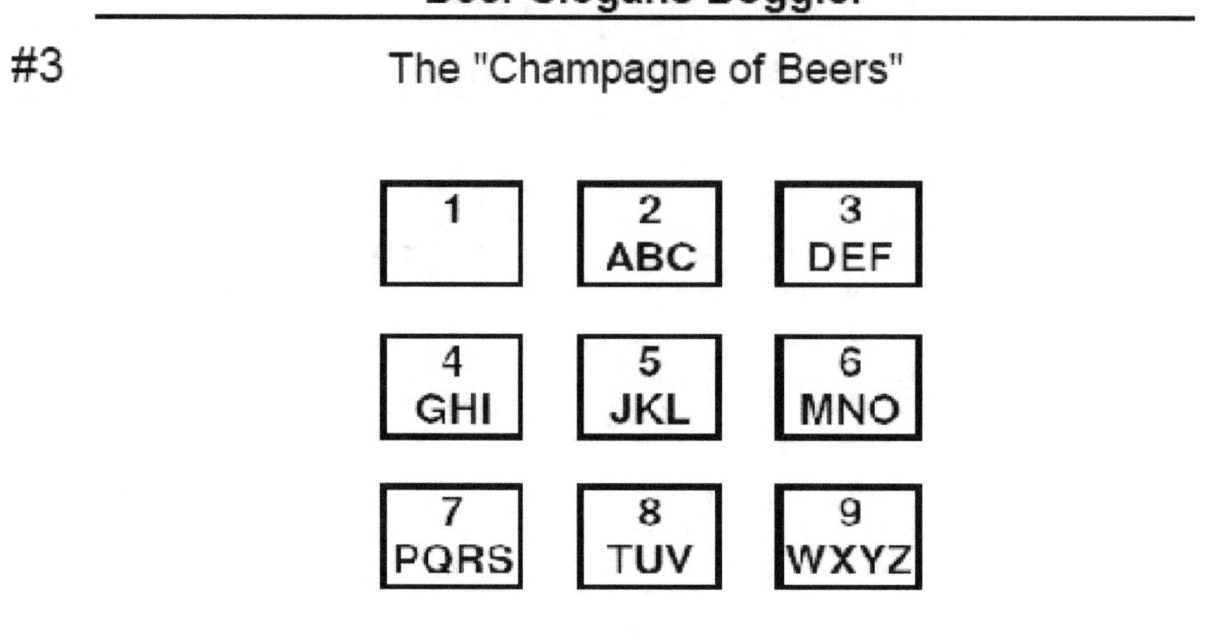

M
— — — — — —   — — — —   — — — —
6 4 5 5 3 7   4 4 4 4   5 4 3 3

#4   "It doesn't get any better than this."

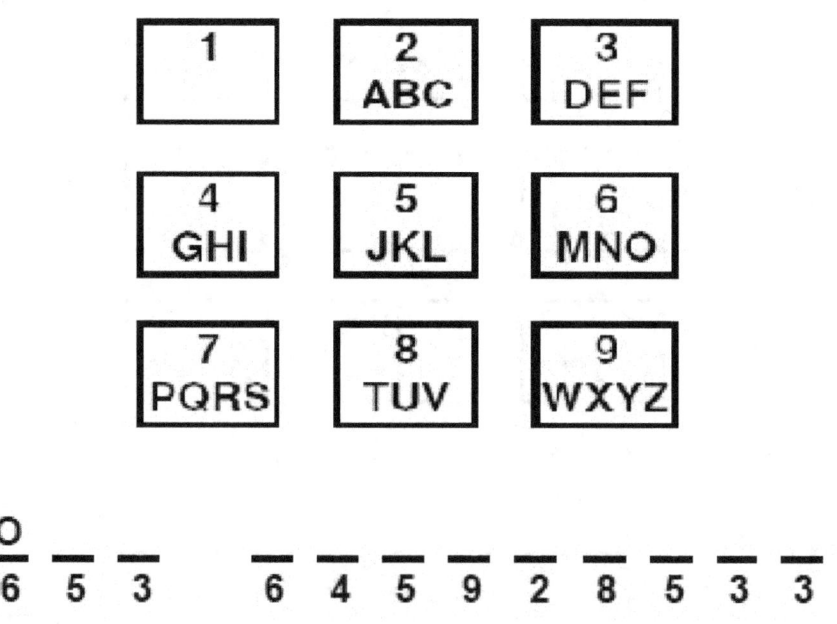

O
— — —   — — — — — — — — —
6 5 3   6 4 5 9 2 8 5 3 3

Code Breakers

Use the telephone dial pad and place the correct letter above each number to break the code and solve the

Beer Slogans Boggler

#5   "The beer that made Milwaukee famous"

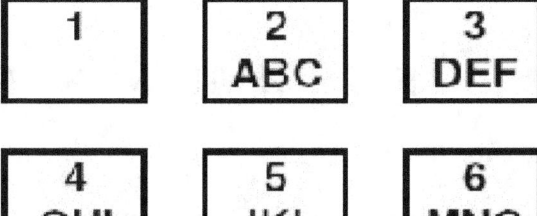

$$\frac{S}{7} \; \frac{}{2} \; \frac{}{4} \; \frac{}{5} \; \frac{}{4} \; \frac{}{8} \; \frac{}{9}$$

#6   "Head for the mountains"

1	2 ABC	3 DEF
4 GHI	5 JKL	6 MNO
7 PQRS	8 TUV	9 WXYZ

$$\frac{B}{2} \; \frac{}{8} \; \frac{}{7} \; \frac{}{2} \; \frac{}{4}$$

Code Breakers - Answers
Beer Lovers' Puzzler

#1 B E N J A M I N F R A N K L I N

#2 A R C H I E B U N K E R

#3 D U F F

#4 C O O R S

#5 S H O T Z

#6 N O R M A N D C L I F F

Code Breakers - Answers
Beer Slogans Boggler

#1   M I L L E R   L I G H T

#2   H E I N E K E N

#3   M I L L E R   H I G H   L I F E

#4   O L D   M I L W A U K E E

#5   S C H L I T Z

#6   B U S C H

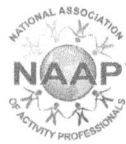 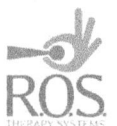

Budget and Time-Saver Activities

As caregivers, our time and finances can often be strained and stretched to the limit. With that in mind, R.O.S. Therapy Systems has designed activity lesson plans that are easy on the budget and use common household items that are readily available from grocery stores or dollar stores.

Activities are not just playing Bingo. It can be anything! Here are some general activity suggestions that can help you get started and do not cost any money.

Around the House Activities

- Making the bed

- Folding laundry items such as napkins or towels

- Reading the newspaper

- Setting the table

- Watching a favorite television game show or program

- Having a conversation

Please remember that as a caregiver, you should be present at all times. No matter how simple YOU think an activity may be, it may be a challenge for the person you are working with, and they may need assistance or some type of verbal cue. If you have designed an activity on your own or used one of the general suggestions above, please use an Activity Lesson Plan form so that all caregivers may see it. For continuity, they will need to access the notes of any verbal cues or assistance which may have been required or given for the participant to enjoy the activity.